How to Control Your Blood Sugar

Rebecca L.

Contents

Introduction:Understanding Blood Sugar

Overview: The Vital Role of Blood Sugar in Human Health

Blood sugar, scientifically known as blood glucose, is a fundamental component of our body's intricate metabolic system. It serves as the primary fuel source for our cells, powering everything from basic cellular functions to complex cognitive processes. This simple sugar, derived primarily from the carbohydrates we consume, circulates in our bloodstream, ready to be utilized by our body's tissues and organs.

The importance of maintaining healthy blood sugar levels cannot be overstated. When blood glucose levels are well-regulated, our bodies function optimally. We experience stable energy levels, clear thinking, and overall well-being. However, when blood sugar levels become imbalanced – either too high or too low – it can lead to a cascade of health issues.

In recent years, the prevalence of blood sugar-related disorders, particularly diabetes and prediabetes, has risen dramatically worldwide. This increase is largely attributed to modern lifestyle factors such as sedentary behavior, poor dietary habits, and increased stress levels. According to the World Health Organization, the number of people with diabetes has risen from 108 million in 1980 to 422 million in 2014, and this number continues to grow.

Diabetes, a condition characterized by chronically elevated blood sugar levels, can lead to severe complications if left unmanaged. These include cardiovascular disease, kidney damage, nerve damage, and vision problems. Prediabetes, a precursor to type 2 diabetes, affects millions more and serves as a warning sign of potential future health issues.

Given these alarming trends, understanding how to control blood sugar has become more critical than ever. It's not just a concern for those diagnosed with diabetes or prediabetes; maintaining healthy blood sugar levels is crucial for everyone's long-term health and vitality.

This book aims to provide a comprehensive guide to blood sugar management. We'll explore the science behind blood glucose regulation, the factors that influence it, and practical strategies for maintaining healthy levels. From nutrition and exercise to stress management and the latest technological advancements, we'll cover all aspects of blood sugar control.

By gaining a deeper understanding of blood sugar and how to manage it effectively, readers will be empowered to take control of their health, potentially preventing or managing diabetes, and improving their overall quality of life. Whether you're dealing with a diagnosed condition or simply seeking to optimize your health, the knowledge and strategies presented in this book will serve as invaluable tools in your journey towards better health and well-being.

Remember, maintaining healthy blood sugar levels is not just about preventing disease – it's about feeling your best, having sustained energy throughout the day, and setting the foundation for a long, healthy life. Let's embark on this journey to understand and master the art of blood sugar control.

Chapter 1: The Science of Blood Sugar

What is Glucose?

Glucose is a simple sugar that is a primary energy source for the body's cells. It is derived from the foods we eat, particularly carbohydrates. When we consume food, our digestive system breaks down carbohydrates into glucose, which then enters the bloodstream.

The Role of Insulin and Other Hormones

Insulin is a hormone produced by the pancreas that allows cells to absorb glucose from the bloodstream for energy or storage. When blood sugar levels rise after eating, the pancreas releases insulin to help lower blood sugar levels by facilitating the uptake of glucose into cells.

Other hormones, such as glucagon, growth hormone, and cortisol, also play roles in blood sugar regulation. Glucagon, for example, works in opposition to insulin by raising blood sugar levels when they are too low.

Normal Blood Sugar Ranges

Normal fasting blood sugar levels typically range from 70 to 99 mg/dL. After eating, blood sugar levels can rise but should generally stay below 140 mg/dL. Consistently high or low blood sugar levels can indicate underlying health issues that need to be addressed.

The Impact of High and Low Blood Sugar

High blood sugar (hyperglycemia) can lead to various health problems, including diabetes, cardiovascular disease, and nerve damage. Symptoms of hyperglycemia include frequent urination, increased thirst, and fatigue.

Low blood sugar (hypoglycemia) can cause symptoms such as shakiness, sweating, confusion, and in severe cases, loss of consciousness. It is crucial to manage blood sugar levels to avoid these complications.

Chapter 2: Factors Affecting Blood Sugar Levels

Diet and Its Impact on Blood Sugar

The food we eat has a direct impact on our blood sugar levels. Carbohydrates, in particular, are broken down into glucose and have the most significant effect on blood sugar. Simple carbohydrates, such as sugary snacks and white bread, can cause rapid spikes in blood sugar, while complex carbohydrates, like whole grains and vegetables, lead to more gradual increases.

The Role of Exercise in Blood Sugar Control

Physical activity helps lower blood sugar levels by increasing insulin sensitivity and allowing cells to use glucose more effectively. Both aerobic exercises (like walking, running, and cycling) and strength training (like weightlifting) can be beneficial.

Stress and Its Effect on Glucose Levels

Stress triggers the release of hormones such as cortisol and adrenaline, which can raise blood sugar levels. Chronic stress can lead to prolonged periods of elevated blood sugar, increasing the risk of developing diabetes.

Sleep and Its Relationship with Blood Sugar

Poor sleep quality and insufficient sleep can negatively affect blood sugar levels. Sleep deprivation can lead to insulin resistance, making it harder for the body to regulate blood sugar effectively.

Medications That Can Affect Blood Sugar

Certain medications, including steroids, beta-blockers, and some antidepressants, can impact blood sugar levels. It is essential to be aware of these potential effects and work with a healthcare provider to manage them.

Chapter 3: Nutrition for Balanced Blood Sugar

Understanding Macronutrients: Carbohydrates, Proteins, and Fats

Each macronutrient affects blood sugar differently. Carbohydrates have the most significant impact, as they are broken down into glucose. Proteins and fats have a more gradual effect on blood sugar and can help stabilize levels when included in meals.

The Glycemic Index and Glycemic Load

The glycemic index (GI) measures how quickly a food raises blood sugar levels. Foods with a high GI cause rapid spikes, while those with a low GI lead to slower increases. Glycemic load (GL) considers both the GI and the carbohydrate content of a food, providing a more comprehensive picture of its impact on blood sugar.

Fiber and Its Role in Blood Sugar Control

Fiber, particularly soluble fiber, can help regulate blood sugar levels by slowing the absorption of glucose. Foods high in fiber, such as fruits, vegetables, and whole grains, are beneficial for maintaining stable blood sugar.

Meal Planning for Stable Blood Sugar

Creating balanced meals that include a mix of carbohydrates, proteins, and fats can help maintain stable blood sugar levels. Eating smaller, more frequent meals throughout the day can also prevent large fluctuations in blood sugar.

Superfoods That Help Regulate Blood Sugar

Certain foods, such as leafy greens, berries, nuts, and seeds, have been shown to help regulate blood sugar levels. Incorporating these superfoods into your diet can provide additional benefits for blood sugar control.

Chapter 4: Exercise and Blood Sugar Management

How Different Types of Exercise Affect Blood Sugar

Different types of exercise can have varying effects on blood sugar levels. Aerobic exercises, such as walking, running, and swimming, can help lower blood sugar by increasing insulin sensitivity. Strength training exercises, like weightlifting, can also improve insulin sensitivity and build muscle mass, which helps the body use glucose more effectively.

Creating an Exercise Plan for Blood Sugar Control

Developing a personalized exercise plan that includes a mix of aerobic and strength training exercises can be beneficial for blood sugar management. Aim for at least 150 minutes of moderate-intensity aerobic exercise per week, along with two or more days of strength training.

Precautions for Exercising with Diabetes

When exercising with diabetes, it's essential to take certain precautions to avoid complications. Monitor blood sugar levels before, during, and after exercise to ensure they remain within a safe range. Stay hydrated, wear appropriate footwear, and carry a source of fast-acting glucose in case of hypoglycemia.

Monitoring Blood Sugar Before, During, and After Exercise

Regularly monitoring blood sugar levels around exercise can help you understand how your body responds to different types of physical activity. This information can be used to adjust your exercise routine and dietary intake to maintain stable blood sugar levels.

Chapter 5: Stress Management and Blood Sugar

The Physiological Link Between Stress and Blood Sugar

Stress triggers the release of hormones such as cortisol and adrenaline, which can raise blood sugar levels. Chronic stress can lead to prolonged periods of elevated blood sugar, increasing the risk of developing diabetes and other health issues.

Stress Reduction Techniques: Meditation, Deep Breathing, Yoga

Practicing stress reduction techniques such as meditation, deep breathing, and yoga can help lower blood sugar levels by reducing the impact of stress hormones. These practices promote relaxation and can improve overall well-being.

The Importance of Adequate Sleep for Blood Sugar Control

Getting enough quality sleep is essential for maintaining healthy blood sugar levels. Sleep deprivation can lead to insulin resistance and higher blood sugar levels. Aim for 7-9 hours of sleep per night and practice good sleep hygiene to improve sleep quality.

Developing Healthy Coping Mechanisms

Finding healthy ways to cope with stress, such as engaging in hobbies, spending time with loved ones, and practicing mindfulness, can help reduce the impact of stress on blood sugar levels. Avoid unhealthy coping mechanisms, such as overeating or consuming alcohol, which can negatively affect blood sugar.

Chapter 6: Monitoring and Tracking Blood Sugar

Different Methods of Blood Sugar Testing

There are various methods for testing blood sugar levels, including fingerstick tests with a glucose meter and continuous glucose monitoring (CGM) systems. Each method has its advantages and can be used to track blood sugar levels effectively.

How to Use a Glucose Meter Effectively

Using a glucose meter involves pricking the finger to obtain a small blood sample, which is then placed on a test strip and inserted into the meter. The meter provides a reading of the blood sugar level. It's essential to follow the manufacturer's instructions and maintain the meter and test strips properly.

Continuous Glucose Monitoring Systems

CGMs provide real-time blood sugar readings throughout the day and night by using a small sensor inserted under the skin. These systems can help identify patterns and trends in blood sugar levels, allowing for more precise management.

Keeping a Blood Sugar Log and Analyzing Trends

Maintaining a blood sugar log can help track levels over time and identify patterns related to diet, exercise, stress, and other factors. Analyzing these trends can provide valuable insights for adjusting lifestyle and treatment plans to maintain stable blood sugar levels.

Chapter 7: Medications and Blood Sugar Control

Introduction

Medications play a crucial role in managing blood sugar levels, especially for individuals with diabetes. This chapter provides an in-depth look at various pharmaceutical options, their mechanisms of action, and how to use them effectively in conjunction with lifestyle changes.

Types of Diabetes Medications

1. Oral Medications

Metformin:
Metformin is often the first-line treatment for type 2 diabetes. It works by reducing glucose production in the liver and improving the body's sensitivity to insulin. Metformin is generally well-tolerated, but some people

may experience gastrointestinal side effects such as nausea and diarrhea.

Sulfonylureas:
These medications stimulate the pancreas to produce more insulin. Common sulfonylureas include glipizide and glyburide. They are effective in lowering blood sugar but can cause hypoglycemia (low blood sugar) and weight gain.

DPP-4 Inhibitors:
DPP-4 inhibitors, such as sitagliptin and saxagliptin, help increase insulin production and reduce glucagon secretion. They are generally well-tolerated and have a low risk of causing hypoglycemia.

SGLT2 Inhibitors:
SGLT2 inhibitors, like canagliflozin and dapagliflozin, work by helping the kidneys remove excess glucose through urine. They can aid in weight loss but may increase the risk of urinary tract infections and dehydration.

2. Injectable Medications

GLP-1 Receptor Agonists:

These medications, including exenatide and liraglutide, slow digestion, promote satiety, and stimulate insulin production. They are effective in lowering blood sugar and promoting weight loss but can cause gastrointestinal side effects.

Insulin Therapy:
Insulin is essential for individuals with type 1 diabetes and may be necessary for those with type 2 diabetes. There are various types of insulin, including rapid-acting, short-acting, intermediate-acting, and long-acting. Insulin can be administered using syringes, pens, or pumps.

Combination Therapies
Combining different medications can enhance blood sugar control. For example, a combination of metformin and a DPP-4 inhibitor can provide better glycemic control than either medication alone. Your healthcare provider will help determine the best combination based on your individual needs.

Medication Management

Adherence:

Taking medications as prescribed is crucial for effective blood sugar management. Strategies to improve adherence include setting reminders, using pill organizers, and incorporating medication into your daily routine.

Side Effects:
Understanding potential side effects and how to manage them is essential. For example, taking metformin with food can reduce gastrointestinal discomfort. Always consult your healthcare provider if you experience adverse effects.

Personalized Medicine in Diabetes
Emerging trends in personalized diabetes treatment focus on tailoring medications to individual genetic profiles. This approach aims to optimize efficacy and minimize side effects. Ongoing research in this field holds promise for more precise diabetes management.

Conclusion

Medications are a vital component of blood sugar management, especially for individuals with diabetes. By understanding the different types of medications, their mechanisms of action, and how to manage them effectively, you can take an active role in your treatment plan. Always work closely with your healthcare provider to ensure your medication regimen is tailored to your specific needs.

Chapter 8: Lifestyle Strategies for Long-Term Blood Sugar Management

Introduction

Long-term blood sugar management requires a holistic approach that integrates various lifestyle strategies. The following are key areas of focus to help you maintain stable blood sugar levels and improve your overall quality of life.

Creating and Maintaining Healthy Habits

Establishing a Routine:

Consistency is key to managing blood sugar levels. Establish a routine for meals, exercise, and medication. Set realistic goals, track your progress, and reward yourself for milestones achieved.

Making Lifestyle Changes Stick:

Adopting new habits can be challenging. Use strategies such as setting specific, achievable goals, breaking larger goals into smaller steps, and seeking support from friends and family.

The Importance of Consistency in Diet and Exercise

Diet:
A balanced diet is crucial for blood sugar control. Focus on whole foods, including vegetables, fruits, lean proteins, and whole grains. Avoid refined carbohydrates and sugary snacks. Understanding the glycemic index and carbohydrate counting can help you make informed food choices.

Exercise:
Regular physical activity helps stabilize blood sugar levels. Aim for at least 150 minutes of moderate-intensity aerobic exercise per week, along with strength training exercises. Find activities you enjoy to maintain motivation and vary your routine to keep it interesting.

Regular Health Check-ups and Screenings

Ongoing Medical Supervision:
Regular check-ups with your healthcare provider are essential for monitoring your blood sugar levels and overall health. Schedule routine screenings such as HbA1c tests, eye exams, and foot exams to detect and prevent complications.

Recommended Frequency:
Discuss with your healthcare provider the recommended frequency of various health checks. For example, HbA1c tests are typically done every 3 to 6 months, while eye exams and foot exams may be annual.

Building a Support System

Involving Family and Friends:
Educate your loved ones about your condition and how they can support you. Involving them in your diabetes management can provide emotional support and practical assistance.

Support Groups:
Joining support groups or online communities can provide additional encouragement and share experiences with others facing similar challenges.

Managing Stress

Stress Reduction Techniques:
Stress can negatively impact blood sugar levels. Practice stress reduction techniques such as meditation, yoga, and deep breathing exercises. These practices promote relaxation and improve overall well-being.

Understanding the Stress-Blood Sugar Link:
Stress triggers the release of hormones like cortisol, which can raise blood sugar levels. By managing stress, you can help keep your blood sugar levels stable.

Sleep and Blood Sugar Management

Quality Sleep:
Getting enough quality sleep is vital for blood sugar control. Aim for 7-9 hours of sleep per night. Poor sleep can lead to insulin resistance and higher blood sugar levels.

Improving Sleep Hygiene:
Establish a regular sleep schedule, create a restful environment, and avoid stimulants like caffeine before bedtime. Practice relaxation techniques to improve sleep quality.

Continuous Learning and Staying Informed

Ongoing Education:
Stay informed about new research and treatments for diabetes management. Utilize reputable resources such as websites, books, and organizations that offer the latest information and support.

Resources:

We provide a list of recommended resources for ongoing diabetes education, including websites, books, and support organizations.

Planning for the Future

Setting Long-Term Health Goals:
Establishing long-term health goals helps maintain focus and motivation. Set achievable objectives and regularly review and adjust them as needed.

Preparing for Potential Complications:
Proactive management and regular monitoring can help prevent complications. Work with your healthcare provider to develop a plan for addressing potential issues.

Conclusion

By focusing on these key areas, you can develop a comprehensive, sustainable approach to long-term blood sugar management. Integrating these strategies into your daily life will help you maintain stable blood sugar levels, prevent complications, and improve your overall quality of life. Remember, managing blood sugar

is a lifelong journey, and staying informed, consistent,
and proactive is essential for success.

References

1. World Health Organization (WHO). Diabetes. WHO media centre, 2006.

2. National Diabetes Information Clearinghouse. National Diabetes Statistics. 2005.

3. Stratton IM, Adler AI, Neil HA, et al. Association of glycaemia with macrovascular and microvascular complications of type 2 diabetes (UKPDS 35): prospective observational study. BMJ. 2000;321:405–12.

4. American Heart Association. Life's Essential 8 - How to Manage Blood Sugar Fact Sheet. heart.org.

5. Registered Nurses' Association of Ontario. Getting to know your diabetes: Reference Guide for People with Diabetes. RNAO.ca.

6. Inchauspe J. Glucose Revolution. (Book)

7. Bryson B. The Body: A Guide for Occupants. (Book)

8. William A. Medical Medium Liver Rescue. (Book)

9. Fung J. The Obesity Code. (Book)

10. Li WW. Eat to Beat Disease. (Book)

11. Mayo Clinic. Diabetes - Diagnosis and treatment. mayoclinic.org.

www.ingramcontent.com/pod-product-compliance
Lightning Source LLC
Chambersburg PA
CBHW050757250726

48662CB00005B/2264